KETO RECIPES

A BEGINNER'S GUIDE TO
KETOGENIC DIET STEP-BY-STEP

BY MARISA BROWN

Table of Contents

1. FRITTATA WITH FRESH SPINACH

BREAKFAST

INGREDIENTS:

- 5 OUNCES. DICED FRANCIS BACON OR CHORIZO
- 2 TBSP BUTTER
- 8 OUNCES. (7½ CUPS) CLEAN SPINACH
- 8 EGGS
- 1 CUP HEAVY WHIPPING CREAM
- 5 OZ. (1¼ CUPS) CHEDDAR CHEESE, SHREDDED
- SALT AND PEPPER

INSTRUCTIONS:

1. Preheat the oven to 350°F (175°C). Grease a 9x9 baking dish or person ramekins.
2. Fry the publisher 1st baron verulam in butter on medium warmth till crispy. Upload the spinach and stir till wilted. Do away with the pan from the heat and set aside.
3. Whisk the eggs and cream collectively and pour into baking dish or in ramekins.
4. Add the Baron Verulam, spinach and cheese on top and place within the middle of the oven. Bake for 25 to 30 minutes or until set in the middle and golden brown on top.

2. FRIED CHICKEN

LUNCH

INGREDIENTS:

FOR THE CHICKEN

- 6 BONE IN, PORES AND SKIN ON CHOOK BREASTS (APPROXIMATELY FOUR LBS.)
- KOSHER SALT
- FRESHLY FLOOR BLACK PEPPER
- 2 LARGE EGGS
- 1/2 C. HEAVY CREAM
- THREE/FOUR C. ALMOND FLOUR
- 1 1/2 C. FINELY CRUSHED RED MEAT RINDS
- 1/2 C. FRESHLY GRATED PARMESAN
- 1 TSP. GARLIC POWDER
- 1/2 TSP. PAPRIKA

INSTRUCTIONS:

1. Preheat oven to 400° and line a large baking sheet with parchment paper. Pat chook dry with paper towels and season with salt and pepper.
2. In a shallow bowl whisk collectively eggs and heavy cream. In another shallow bowl, integrate almond flour, pork rinds, Parmesan, garlic powder, and paprika. Season with salt and pepper.
3. Running one by one, dip chook in egg aggregate after which in almond flour combination, pressing to coat. Place fowl on organized baking sheet.
4. Bake till chicken is golden and internal temperature reaches one hundred sixty five, about forty five mins.

5. Meanwhile, make dipping sauce: In a medium bowl, integrate mayonnaise and hot sauce. Add more hot sauce relying on favored spiciness stage.
6. Serve chook heat with dipping sauce.

3. MAC AND CHEESE

LUNCH

INGREDIENTS:

FOR THE MAC & CHEESE

BUTTER, FOR BAKING DISH
2 MEDIUM HEADS CAULIFLOWER, CUT INTO FLORETS
2 TBSP. GREATER to VIRGIN OLIVE OIL
KOSHER SALT
1 C. HEAVY CREAM
6 OZ.. CREAM CHEESE, CUT INTO CUBES
4 C. SHREDDED CHEDDAR
2 C. SHREDDED MOZZARELLA
1 TBSP. WARM SAUCE (OPTIONALLY AVAILABLE)
FRESHLY FLOOR BLACK PEPPER

FOR THE TOPPING

4 OZ. RED MEAT RINDS, BEATEN
1/4 C. FRESHLY GRATED PARMESAN
1 TBSP. GREATER to VIRGIN OLIVE OIL
2 TBSP. FRESHLY CHOPPED PARSLEY, FOR GARNISH

INSTRUCTIONS:

1. Preheat oven to 375° and butter a 9 "x 13" baking dish. In a large bowl, toss cauliflower with 2 tablespoons oil and season with salt. Unfold cauliflower onto big baking sheets and roast until tender and gently golden, approximately 40 mins.
2. Meanwhile, in a large pot over medium heat, warmth cream. Bring as much as a simmer, then decrease heat to low and stir in cheeses until melted. Eliminate from warmness, upload hot sauce if using and season with salt and pepper, then fold in roasted cauliflower. Flavor and season more if wished.
3. Transfer combination to prepared baking dish. In a medium bowl stir to mix pork rinds, Parmesan, and oil. Sprinkle mixture in a fair layer over cauliflower and cheese.
4. Bake till golden, 15 minutes. If favored, turn oven to broil to toast topping further, approximately 2 mins.
5. Garnish with parsley earlier than serving.

4. MEATBALLS

DINNER

INGREDIENTS:

- 1 HALF LB. GROUND BEEF (80/20)
- 1 TSP. OREGANO
- HALF OF TSP. ITALIAN SEASONING
- 2 TSP. MINCED GARLIC
- HALF OF TSP. ONION POWDER
- 3 TBSP. TOMATO PASTE
- 3 TBSP. FLAXSEED MEAL
- 2 LARGE EGGS
- HALF CUP OLIVES, SLICED
- 1/2 CUP MOZZARELLA CHEESE
- 1 TSP. WORCESTERSHIRE SAUCE
- SALT AND PEPPER TO TASTE

INSTRUCTIONS:

1. In a big mixing bowl, add your ground beef, oregano, Italian seasoning, garlic and onion powder. Mix together properly the usage of your palms.
2. Upload your eggs, tomato paste, flaxseed, and Worcestershire to the beef and mix together again.
3. In the end, slice your olives into small pieces and add this for your meat in conjunction with the shredded mozzarella cheese. Mix the entirety together well.
4. Preheat your oven to 400F after which begin to form the meatballs. You must become with approximately 20 meatballs in total. Lay those on a foil blanketed cookie sheet.

5. Bake the meatballs for 16 to 20 minutes or until the favored carried outness is reached.
6. Serve up with a easy spinach salad below and drizzle with excess fat from the cookie sheet.

o This makes 4 servings of Italian crammed Meatballs. Every serving comes out to be 594 cals, 44.8g fat, 3.8g carbs, and 36.8g protein.

5. CHICKEN PARMESAN
DINNER

INGREDIENTS:

• THREE SMALL CHOOK BREASTS
• SALT AND PEPPER TO FLAVOR
• 1 CUP MOZZARELLA CHEESE

THE COATING

• 2.5 OUNCES. PORK RINDS
• 1/FOUR CUP FLAXSEED MEAL
• 1/2 CUP PARMESAN CHEESE
• 1 TSP. OREGANO
• HALF TSP. SALT
• HALF TSP. PEPPER
• 1/FOUR TSP. PINK PEPPER FLAKES
• HALF OF TSP. GARLIC
• 2 TSP. PAPRIKA
• 1 LARGE EGG
• 1 HALF OF TSP. FOWL BROTH
• 1/4 CUP OLIVE OIL

THE SAUCE

• 1/FOUR CUP OLIVE OIL

- 1 CUP RAO'S TOMATO SAUCE
- 1/2 TSP. GARLIC
- HALF TSP. OREGANO
- SALT AND PEPPER TO TASTE

INSTRUCTIONS:

1. Grind up pork rinds, flaxseed meal, parmesan cheese, and spices in a food processor.
2. Slice chicken breasts in 1/2 or in thirds and pound them out into cutlets. Season to taste.
3. In a separate field to the coating, crack and egg and whisk with 1 half tsp. Bird broth.
4. In a saucepan, integrate all elements for the sauce and whisk together. Let this cook for at least 20 mins at the same time as you are making the hen.
5. Bread all fowl cutlets by way of dipping into egg mixture, then dipping into the coating combination. Set aside on a chunk of foil.
6. Warmth 2 tbsp. Olive oil in a pan and fry up each piece of chicken 2 at a time.
7. Upload more oil as needed (I used 1/four cup in general).
8. Set portions of bird right into a casserole dish, upload sauce on top, and then sprinkle with 1 cup of mozzarella cheese. Bake at 400F for 10 minutes or until cheese is excellent and melted.
9. Serve up with a few broccoli and olives at the facet! You could as an alternative serve up 1 chook cutlet with olives and broccoli for a smaller serving length.

- This makes four servings of bird Parmesan.each serving comes out to be 646 cals, 46.8g fat, 4g carbs, and forty 9.3g protein.

6. LEMON RASPBERRY POPSICLES

Snacks

INGREDIENTS:

- 100G RASPBERRIES
- JUICE HALF LEMON
- 1/4 CUP COCONUT OIL
- 1 CUP COCONUT MILK (FROM THE CARTON)
- 1/4 CUP BITTER CREAM
- 1/4 CUP HEAVY CREAM • HALF OF TSP. GUAR GUM
- 20 DROPS LIQUID STEVIA

INSTRUCTIONS:

1. Add all components right into a container and use an immersion blender to mixture the aggregate collectively.
2. Continue mixing until the raspberries are absolutely jumbled together with the rest of the elements.
3. Pressure the mixture, making sure to discard all raspberry seeds. I tried mak to ing a batch with the seeds still in, and they started out to irritate my tongue as i used to be ingesting it.
4. Pour the combination into molds. I use this mould for my popsicles. Set the pop to sicles within the freezer for no less than 2 hours.
5. Run the mildew below hot water to dislodge the popsicles. 6. Serve and eat on every occasion you want!

o   This makes a total of 6 Raspberry Lemon Popsicles each popsicle comes out to be 151 cals, 16g fats, 2g carbs, and 0.5g protein.

7. FAT NEPOLITAN BOMBS

Snacks

INGREDIENTS:

- HALF CUP BUTTER
- 1/2 CUP COCONUT OIL
- HALF OF CUP BITTER CREAM
- 1/2 CUP CREAM CHEESE
- 2 TBSP. ERYTHRITOL
- 25 DROPS LIQUID STEVIA
- 2 TBSP. COCOA POWDER
- 1 TSP. VANILLA EXTRACT
- 2 MEDIUM STRAWBERRIES

INSTRUCTIONS:

1. In a bowl, integrate butter, coconut oil, bitter cream, cream cheese, erythritol, and liquid stevia.
2. The usage of an immersion blender, mixture collectively the elements right into a easy combination.
3. Divide the combination into three one of a kind bowls. Add cocoa powder to 1 bowl, strawberries to any other bowl, and vanilla to the final bowl.
4. Mix together all of the substances again the use of an immersion blender. Sep to arate the chocolate aggregate right into a field with a spout.
5. Pour chocolate combination into fats bomb mold. Location in freezer for 30 minutes, then repeat with the vanilla combination.
6. Freeze vanilla aggregate for half to hour, then repeat process with strawberry mixture. Freeze again for at least 1 hour.
7. When they're absolutely frozen, put off from the fat bomb molds.

- This makes a total of 24 Neapolitan fats Bombs. each fats bomb comes out to be 102 cals, 10.9g fat, 0.4g carbs, and 0.6g protein.

8. Coconut orange fat bomb

Snack

INGREDIENTS:

- HALF CUP COCONUT OIL
- HALF OF CUP HEAVY WHIPPING CREAM
- 4 OUNCES. CREAM CHEESE
- 1 TSP. ORANGE VANILLA MIO • 10 DROPS LIQUID STEVIA

INSTRUCTIONS:

1. degree out coconut oil, heavy cream, and cream cheese.
2. Use an immersion blender to mixture collectively all of the elements. if you're having a tough time mixing the elements, you can microwave them for 30 seconds to at least one minute to soften them up.
3. add Orange Vanilla Mio and liquid stevia into the aggregate and mix together with a spoon.
4. unfold the combination right into a silicone tray (Mine is an first rate Avenger's Ice cube Tray) and freeze for two to three hours.
5. once hardened, do away with from the silicone tray and shop in the freezer. enjoy!

- This makes a complete of 10 Coconut Orange Creamsicle fats Bombs every fats bomb comes out to be 176 cals, 20g fat, 0.7g carbs, and 0.8g protein.

○

9. PIZZA FAT BOMBS

SNACKS

INGREDEINTS:

FOUR OZ. CREAM CHEESE
14 SLICES PEPPERONI
8 PITTED BLACK OLIVES
2 TBSP. SOLAR DRIED TOMATO

PESTO

2 TBSP. SPARKLING BASIL, CHOPPED
SALT AND PEPPER TO TASTE

INSTRUCTIONS:

1. Dice pepperoni and olives into small portions.
2. Blend together basil, tomato pesto, and cream cheese.
3. Upload the olives and pepperoni into the cream cheese and mix again.
4. Form into balls, then garnish with pepperoni, basil, and olive.

o This makes a total of 6 Pizza fat Bombs.each fat bomb comes out to be one hundred ten cals, 10.5g fat, 1.3g carbs, and 2.3g protein.

10. CHOCOLATE PEANUT BUTTER Snack

INGREDIENTS:

- HALF OF CUP COCONUT OIL
- 1/4 CUP COCOA POWDER
- 4 TBSP. PB SUIT POWDER
- 6 TBSP. SHELLED HEMP SEEDS
- 2 TBSP. HEAVY CREAM
- 1 TSP. VANILLA EXTRACT
- 28 DROPS LIQUID STEVIA
- 1/4 CUP UNSWEETENED SHREDDED COCONUT

INSTRUCTIONS:

1. Blend collectively all the dry substances with the coconut oil. It may take a piece of labor, however it'll sooner or later change into a paste.
2. Upload heavy cream, vanilla, and liquid stevia. Mix once more until the whole lot is blended and slightly creamy.
3. Degree out unsweetened shredded coconut directly to a plate.
4. Roll balls out using your hand and then roll in the unsweetened shred to ded coconut. Lay on to a baking tray included in parchment paper. Set inside the freezer for about 20 minutes.
5. Revel in!

- This makes a total of eight No Bake Chocolate Peanut Butter fat Bombs.every fats bomb comes out to be 208 cals, 20g fats, 0.8g carbs, and 4.4g protein.

11.   TORTILLA CHIPS

Snacks

INGREDIENTS:

TORTILLA CHIPS

- 6 FLAXSEED TORTILLAS (RECIPE HERE)
- OIL FOR DEEP FRYING,
- (~THREE TBSP. ABSORBED OIL)
- SALT AND PEPPER TO FLAVOR

OPTIONALTOPPINGS

- DICED JALAPENO
- CLEAN SALSA
- SHREDDED CHEESE
- COMPLETE FAT SOUR CREAM

INSTRUCTIONS:

1. Make the flaxseed tortilla's the use of this recipe. I get 6 total tortillas whilst the usage of a tortilla press.
2. Reduce the tortillas into chip to sized slices. I were given 6 out of every tortilla.
3. Warmth the deep fryer. Once ready, lay out the portions of tortilla within the basket.
4. You may fry 4 to 6 portions at a time.
5. Fry for approximately 1 to 2 mins, then flip. Hold to fry for every other 1 to 2 mins on the other aspect.
6. Cast off from the fryer and place on paper towels to cool. Season with salt and pepper to taste.
7. Serve with toppings of desire!

○ This makes a total of 36 Keto Tortilla Chips. Every chip is about 27 cals, 3.1g fats, 0.04g Carbs (almost zero), and 0.9g protein.

12.   J
alapeno fat bombs

SNACKS

INGREDIENTS:

- THREE OZ. CREAM CHEESE
- 3 SLICES SIR FRANCIS BACON
- 1 MEDIUM JALAPENO PEPPER
- 1/2 TSP. DRIED PARSLEY
- 1/4 TSP. ONION POWDER
- 1/4 TSP. GARLIC POWDER
- SALT AND PEPPER TO FLAVOR

INSTRUCTIONS:

1. Fry 3 slices of Sir Francis Bacon in a pan until crisp.
2. Put off 1st Baron Beaverbrook from the pan, however keep the ultimate grease for later use. 3. Wait till publisher 1st baron verulam is cooled and crisp.
3. De seed a jalapeno pepper, then dice into small portions.
4. Combine cream cheese, jalapeno, and spices. Season with salt and pep consistent with to flavor.
5. Add the 1st Baron Verulam fat in and mix together until a solid mixture is formed.
6. Collapse publisher 1st baron verulam and set on a plate. Roll cream cheese combination into balls the usage of your hand, then roll the ball into the 1st Baron Beaverbrook.

- This makes a complete of three Jalapeno Popper fats Bombs. each fats bomb comes out to be: 207 cals, 19.3g fats, 1.5g carb, and 4.8g protein
-

13.   CHEESEBURGER MUFFINS
SNACKS

INGREDIENTS:

CHEESEBURGER MUFFIN BUNS

- 1/2 CUP BLANCHED ALMOND FLOUR
- HALF CUP FLAXSEED MEAL
- 1 TSP. BAKING POWDER
- HALF OF TSP. SALT
- 1/4 TSP. PEPPER
- 2 LARGE EGGS
- 1/4 CUP SOUR CREAM

HAMBURGER FILLING

- 16 OZ. FLOOR RED MEAT
- 1/2 TSP. ONION POWDER
- 1/2 TSP. GARLIC POWDER
- 2 TBSP. TOMATO PASTE
- SALT AND PEPPER TO TASTE

TOPPINGS

- HALF OF CUP CHEDDAR CHEESE (~1.FIVE OZ..)
- 18 SLICES TODDLER DILL PICKLES (~1 PICKLE)
- 2 TBSP. REDUCED SUGAR KETCHUP
- 2 TBSP. MUSTARD

INSTRUCTIONS:

1. Measure out the ground beef and region into a warm pan. Season with salt and pepper.
2. Cook dinner red meat till browned on the lowest, the season with onion powder, garlic powder, and tomato paste. Mix collectively and turn off the warmth. You have to be left with "uncommon" (most effective semi to cooked) floor red meat.
3. Blend together the dry ingredients for the truffles and pre to warmness oven to 350f.
4. Add wet elements into the muffin aggregate and mix well.
5. Divide up the aggregate for the muffins into silicone muffin cups. Indent the muffin the usage of your finger or a spoon to give area for the floor red meat. Then, fill every muffin with floor red meat mixture.
6. Bake for 15 to 20 minutes or till cakes are browned slightly at the out of doors.
7. Dispose of from the oven and pinnacle with a few cheese, then broil for an additional 1 to 3 mins.
8. Permit cool for 5 to10 mins, then get rid of from the silicone muffin cups.
9. Serve and revel in! Top with chopped pickles, ketchup, mustard or your favorite condiments!

o This makes nine Keto Cheeseburger muffins. every muffin comes out to be 246 cals, 18.6g fat, 1.9g carbs, and 14.2g protein.

14. PERSONAL PAN PIZZA
SNACKS

INGREDIENTS:

PERSONAL PAN PIZZA DIP

- FOUR OZ. CREAM CHEESE
- 4 CUP SOUR CREAM
- 1/FOUR CUP MAYONNAISE
- HALF CUP MOZZARELLA CHEESE, SHREDDED
- SALT AND PEPPER TO FLAVOR
- HALF CUP RAO'S TOMATO SAUCE
- HALF OF CUP MOZZARELLA CHEESE, SHREDDED
- 1/FOUR CUP PARMESAN CHEESE

PEPPERONI, PEPPERS, & OLIVES

- 6 SLICES PEPPERONI, CHOPPED
- 1 TBSP. GREEN PEPPER, SLICED
- 4 PITTED BLACK OLIVES, SLICED
- HALF OF TSP. ITALIAN SEASONING
- SALT AND PEPPER TO FLAVOR

MUSHROOM AND PEPPERS

- 1 TBSP. GREEN PEPPER, SLICED
- 2 TBSP. BABY BELLA MUSHROOMS, CHOPPED
- 1/2 TSP. ITALIAN SEASONING
- SALT AND PEPPER TO FLAVOR

INSTRUCTIONS:

1. Pre heat oven to 350F. Measure out the cream cheese and microwave for 20 seconds till room temperature.

2. Blend the bitter cream, mayonnaise, and mozzarella cheese into the cream cheese. Season with salt and pepper to taste.
3. Divide the combination among 4 ramekins.
4. Spoon 2 tbsp. Rao's Tomato Sauce over every ramekin and unfold out calmly.
5. Measure out 1/2 cup mozzarella cheese and 1/4 cup parmesan cheese. Sprinkle aggregate over the top of the sauce frivolously, then upload toppings of choice to your personal pan pizza dips.
6. Bake for 18 to 20 minutes or till cheese is effervescent. Remove from the oven and permit cool for a second.
7. Serve with a few scrumptious keto breadsticks or beef rinds!

o Yields four servings of private Pan Pizza Dip.each serving comes out to be:
Pepperoni, Peppers, & Olives: 414 energy, 37.8g fat, four.5g internet Carbs, and 15g Protein. Mushroom and Peppers:349 calories, 31.5g fat, 4g internet Carbs, and 12.5g Protein.

15. CORNDOG MUFFINS
SNACKS

INGREDIENTS:

- HALF OF CUP BLANCHED ALMOND FLOUR
- HALF CUP FLAXSEED MEAL
- 1 TBSP. PSYLLIUM HUSK POWDER
- 3 TBSP. SWERVE SWEETENER
- 1/4 TSP. SALT
- 1/4 TSP. BAKING POWDER
- 1/4 CUP BUTTER, MELTED
- 1 LARGE EGG
- 1/3 CUP SOUR CREAM
- 1/4 CUP COCONUT MILK
- 10 LIT'L SMOKIES (OR THREE HOT PUPPIES)

INSTRUCTIONS:

1. Pre heat oven to 375F. mix together all of the dry components in a bowl. make certain all the elements are properly allotted.
2. add your egg, bitter cream, and butter and then blend nicely.
3. as soon as blended, add the coconut milk and keep combining.
4. Divide the batter up among 20 properly greased mini muffin slots, then reduce the Lit'l Smokies in 1/2 and stick them in the center it doesn't get simpler.
5. you can get a mini muffin tray on amazon.
6. Bake for 12 mins and then broil for 1 to 2 minutes till the tops are lightly browned. feel free to use a fork or your arms to push the portions of warm dog back into the muffin in the event that they rise with the batter.
7. let the cakes cool for a few minutes inside the tray, then dispose of and allow cool on a wire rack.
8. Serve up with some spring onion (optional). you can additionally blend together may additionally onnaise, ketchup, and chili paste to make a candy and highly spiced dipping sauce!

- This makes 20 Keto Corndog muffins. every muffin comes out to be 79 cals, 6.8g fat, zero.7g internet carbs, and 2.4g protein.

16. TROPICAL SMOOTHIE

SNACKS

INGREDIENTS:

- 7 ICE CUBES
- THREE/FOUR CUP UNSWEETENED COCONUT MILK
- 1/4 CUP BITTER CREAM
- 2 TBSP. GOLDEN FLAXSEED MEAL
- 1 TBSP. MCT OIL
- 20 DROPS LIQUID STEVIA
- HALF OF TSP. MANGO EXTRACT
- 1/4 TSP. BLUEBERRY EXTRACT
- 1/4 TSP. BANANA EXTRACT

YOU MAY GET THE EXTRACTS AS A HARD AND FAST ON AMAZON.

INSTRUCTIONS:

1. Placed all the components interior of your blender and wait a few minutes even as the flax meal soaks up some of the moisture. I'm the use of a ninja blender with mini ninja attachment.
2. Mixture on excessive pace for 1 to 2 mins or till consistency is thickened.
3. Pour out on a warm day, sit returned, and enjoy!

- This makes 1 Keto Tropical Smoothie. For the whole lot, it comes out to be 352 cals, 31g fat, 3g carbs, and 5g protein.

17. CUCUMBER SPINACH SMOOTHIE

SNACKS

INGREDIENTS:

- 2 HANDFULS SPINACH
- 2.FIVE OUNCES. CUCUMBER, PEELED AND CUBED
- 7 ICE CUBES
- 1 CUP COCONUT MILK
- (FROM CARTON)
- 12 DROPS LIQUID STEVIA
- 1/4 TSP. XANTHAN GUM
- 1 TO 2 TBSP. MCT OIL

INSTRUCTIONS:

1. This one is outstanding easy to make and you'll have it prepared in just below five mins begin to finish. snatch 2 handfuls of spinach and toss them in a blender, then add 7 ice cubes, 1 cup coconut milk (from the carton), 12 drops stevia, 1/four tsp. xanthan gum, and 1 to 2 tbsp. MCT Oil. Peel the cucumber and dice it, and positioned that over the top. I'm using a ninja blender with the mini to ninja connect to ment and truely love it.
2. combo the shake for 1 to 2 minutes or till all of the substances are properly incor to porated. You'll nonetheless notice little bits of spinach floating around, but you can't flavor them in the texture, so don't fear too much!
3. Pour into a pleasing big glass and take your time playing the refreshingly sweet flavor!

○ This makes 1 total serving of Cucumber Spinach Smoothie. The totals pop out to be 335 cals, 33g fats, 4g carbs, and 3g protein.

18. CINNAMON ROLL POPS

SNACKS

INGREDIENTS:

AS AN AWFUL LOT OR AS LITTLE OF THIS RECI to PE AS YOU WANT: CINNAMON ROLL "OATMEAL"

INSTRUCTIONS:

1. Take something quantity you need of the Cinnamon Roll "Oatmeal" recipe you've got made and stick it inside the blender. Blend it up as lots as you need (or under no circumstances). I feel it enables with the texture and freezing of the very last popsicles.
2. Spoon the combination into your popsicle mold. It takes approximately 1/4 cup to fill every up.
3. The use of your spoon, slide it into and out of the popsicle mildew to get out any air bubbles that can be inner. Ensure that you don't overfill the molds due to the fact the top will stick to them in any other case.
4. Placed the lid on pinnacle of the popsicle molds and slide the popsicle sticks into the slots on the pinnacle. You don't want them to move all of the way to the bottom.
5. Put the popsicle mold into the freezer and permit to freeze absolutely. This can take 3 to four hours (and might live to your freezer so long as you need).
6. Run a hot water bathtub on your sink and submerge the popsicle molds into the new water for 20 to 30 seconds.
7. Take the lid off of the popsicle mold, pulling and wiggling the popsicles as you pull. They need to come out quite without problems. Experience!

○ Serving comes out to 100 cals, 9.4g fats, 0.8g carbs, 2.2g proteins.

19. LAYERED QUESO BLANCO
SNACKS

INGREDIENTS:

- 5 OZ. QUESO BLANCO
- 1 1/2 TBSP. OLIVE OIL
- 2 OZ. OLIVES
- PINCH RED PEPPER FLAKES

INSTRUCTIONS:

1. cur out cheese into cubes, then vicinity in freezer at the same time as you warm up the oil.
2. warmness up the oil in a skillet on medium excessive heat.
3. upload cheese cubes to pan once they're hot and allow to in part melt at the bottom. ok, this is the element wherein I were given a little irritated whilst i used to be setting this together.
4. try to flip the cubes of cheese with a spatula and get as lots browning as possible. as soon as you've got, pass the cheese together and GET MAD! Press it down with a spatula and ensure it all combines together.
5. preserve cooking the cheese, then turn half of the cheese into itself.
6. keep pressing the cheese down, disposing of any excess oil from it.
7. keep flipping and cooking the cheese until a pleasing crust is formed.
8. the use of another spatula, fork, or knife, shape a block with the melting cheese and seal all of the edges off.
9. remove from the pan and allow barely cool.
10. Use a knife to reduce the cheese into cubes. You need it to be warm and nonetheless gooey within the center right here.
11. Serve up with some olive and a pinch of purple pepper flakes.

- I only count 1 tsp. of olive oil inside the macros because that's all i found was absorbed. This got here out to be 525 cals, 43g fat, 2g carbs, and 30g protein.

20.   MAPLE PECAN BARS

SNACKS

INGREDIENTS:

- 2 CUPS PECAN HALVES
- 1 CUP ALMOND FLOUR
- HALF OF CUP GOLDEN FLAXSEED MEAL
- HALF OF CUP UNSWEETENED SHREDDED COCONUT
- HALF CUP COCONUT OIL
- 1/4 CUP "MAPLE SYRUP" (RECIPE RIGHT HERE)
- 1/4 TSP. LIQUID STEVIA (~25 DROPS)

INSTRUCTIONS:

1. Measure out 2 cups of pecan halves and bake for 6 to 8 mins at 350F in the oven. Simply enough to after they begin turning into aromatic.
2. Take away pecans from the oven, then upload to a plastic bag. Use a rolling pin to crush them into chunks. It doesn't remember too much approximately the consistency, but i love to get relatively huge chunks so i will see them within the bars as I eat it.
3. Mix the dry ingredients right into a bowl: 1 cup Almond Flour, 1/2 cup Golden Flaxseed Meal, and half of cup Unsweetened Shredded Coconut.
4. Add the beaten pecans to the bowl and mix together again.
5. Eventually, upload the 1/2 cup Coconut Oil, 1/4 cup "Maple Syrup" (recipe here), and 1/four tsp. Liquid Stevia. Mix this collectively properly until a crumbly dough is for to med.
6. Press the dough into a casserole dish. I am the usage of an 11×7 baking dish for this.

7. Bake for 20 to 25 minutes at 350F, or till the edges are lightly browned.
8. Get rid of from the oven, permit to partially cool, and refrigerate for at the least 1 hour (to cut cleanly).
9. Cut into 12 slices and get rid of the usage of a spatula.

o This makes 12 total servings of Maple Pecan fat Bomb Bars. each serving comes out to be 303 cals, 30.5g fat, 2g carbs, and 4.9g protein.

21. CHIA SEED CRACKERS SNACKS

INGREDIENTS:

- HALF CUP CHIA SEEDS, GROUND • THREE OUNCES. SHREDDED CHEDDAR CHEESE
- 1 1/FOUR CUP ICE WATER
- 2 TBSP. PSYLLIUM HUSK POWDER • 2 TBSP. OLIVE OIL
- 1/4 TSP. XANTHAN GUM
- 1/FOUR TSP. GARLIC POWDER
- 1/FOUR TSP. ONION POWDER • 1/4 TSP. OREGANO
- 1/4 TSP. PAPRIKA
- 1/4 TSP. SALT
- 1/FOUR TSP. PEPPER

INSTRUCTIONS:

1. Preheat oven to 375F. Grind half cup Chia Seeds in a spice grinder. You want a meal like texture.
2. Upload ground Chia Seeds, 2 tbsp. Psyllium Husk Powder, 1/4 tsp. Xanthan Gum, 1/4 tsp. Garlic Powder, 1/four tsp. Onion Powder, 1/4 tsp. Oregano, 1/4 tsp. Paprika, 1/4 tsp. Salt and 1/4 tsp. Pepper to a bowl. Blend this together well.
3. Add 2 tbsp. Olive Oil to the dry elements and blend it together. It must become the consistency of moist sand.
4. Upload 1 1/four cup ice bloodless water to the bowl. Mix it collectively very well. You could need to spend greater time blending it collectively because the chia seeds and psyl to lium take a bit bit of time to take in the water. Maintain blending until a solid dough is fashioned.
5. Grate three oz. Cheddar Cheese and upload it to the bowl.
6. The usage of your arms, knead the dough together. You need it to be enormously dry and no longer sticky by the time you end.
7. Positioned the dough onto a silpat and permit it sit for a couple of minutes.

8. Spread or roll the dough out skinny so that it covers the whole silpat. If you can get it thinner, preserve rolling and keep the extra for a 2d cook.
9. Bake for 30 to 35 minutes inside the oven till cooked.
10. Taken them out of the oven, and at the same time as hot, reduce into man or woman crackers. You can both use the blunt fringe of a knife (don't reduce into the silicone), or a large spatula.
11. Positioned the crackers lower back into the oven for 5 to 7 mins on broil, or till the tops are browned and nicely crisped. Remove from the oven and set on a rack to cool. As they cool, they get greater crisp.
12. Serve up together with your favorite sauces. I'm the usage of my Roasted Garlic Chipotle Aioli.
o   Makes a total of 36 crackers with a little left over dough. according to cracker, these are 31 cals, 2.5g fats, 0.1g carbs, and 1.3g protein.

22.   KETO CHOCOLATE CHUNK COOKIES
SNACKS

INGREDIENTS:

- 1 CUP ALMOND FLOUR
- THREE TBSP. UNFLAVORED WHEY PROTEIN
- 2 TBSP. COCONUT FLOUR
- 2 TBSP. PSYLLIUM HUSK POW to DER
- 8 TBSP. UNSALTED BUTTER
- 2 TSP. BEST VANILLA EXTRACT • 1/FOUR CUP ERYTHRITOL
- 10 DROPS LIQUID STEVIA
- 1/2 TSP. BAKING POWDER
- 1 HUGE EGG
- 5 BARS CHOCOPERFECTION
- (OR OTHER 95%+ COCOA BAR)

INSTRUCTIONS:

1. Preheat the oven to 350F. Then, mix together 1 cup Almond Flour, three tbsp. Unflavored Whey Protein, 2 tbsp. Coconut Flour, 2 tbsp. Psyllium Husk Powder and 1/2 tsp. Baking Powder.
2. the use of a hand mixer, beat eight tbsp. room temperature butter to a light coloration. This ought to take approximately 1 to 2 minutes.
3. add 1/4 cup Erythritol and 10 drops Liquid Stevia to the butter and beat once more.
4. add 1 massive egg and a pair of tsp. excellent Vanilla Extract to the overwhelmed butter and beat again until well combined.
5. Sift dry ingredients over butter and mix again to mix absolutely. make sure there are not any lumps whilst you end.
6. Chop the five bars of Chocoperfection (or other 95%+ Cocoa) and upload to the dough. mix collectively nicely.

7. Roll the dough into a log. Make small markings over the top of the log to make sure steady measurements of cookies.
8. Slice off each piece of dough and roll into a ball. Lay every ball onto a sil pat this is on a baking sheet.
9. using the lowest of a mason jar, lightly press the cookies flat into circles.
10. Bake the cookies for 12 to 15 mins or until a light golden brown shade appears on the edges.
11. allow cool for 5 to10 mins before doing away with from the baking sheet.
12. Serve up with a pleasant glass of coconut or almond milk, and revel in!

○ Makes 16 total Keto Chocolate chunk Cookies.every cookie may have 118 cals, 10.8g fat, 1.6g carbs, and 2.6g protein.

23.   GOAT CHEESE TARTS
SNACKS

INGREDIENTS:

ROASTED TOMATOES

2 MEDIUM TOMATOES, REDUCE INTO 1/4 SLICES
1/4 CUP OLIVE OIL
SALT & PEPPER TO FLAVOR

TART BASE

HALF CUP ALMOND FLOUR
1 TBSP. PSYLLIUM HUSK
2 TBSP. COCONUT FLOUR
5 TBSP. COLD BUTTER, CUBED
1/FOUR TSP. SALT

TART FILLING

HALF MEDIUM ONION, SLICED THIN
THREE OZ.. GOAT CHEESE
2 TBSP. OLIVE OIL
2 TSP. MINCED GARLIC
THREE TSP. FRESH THYME

INSTRUCTIONS:

1. Preheat oven to 425F, then slice 2 medium tomatoes into 1/4 slices. You ought to get at the least 6 slices consistent with tomato.
2. Lay slices on a baking sheet with parchment paper, then drizzle with 1/four cup olive oil and season with salt and pepper to taste. Poke the tomatoes the use of enamel alternatives so that the

juice can run out of the tomatoes and now not motive a "steaming" impact.

3. Bake the tomatoes for 30 to 40 minutes or till they may be roasted and have misplaced most in their juice.
4. Set the tomatoes apart.
5. In a food processor, combine 1/2 cup Almond Flour, 1 tbsp. Psyllium Husk, 2 tbsp. Coconut Flour, and 1/4 tsp. Salt.
6. Dice 5 tbsp. Bloodless Butter and add it to the meals processor also.
7. Slowly pulse the ingredients until a dough starts to form.
8. Press dough into silicone cupcake molds. You need to ensure those layers are pretty thin. Approximately 1/4 1/2 thick.
9. Lessen oven warmth to 350F and bake the brownies at 350F for 17 to 20 mins or till golden brown.
10. Put off truffles from the oven and let cool. Once cooled, turn the silicone cupcake molds the other way up and gently tap the lowest so that the tart dough falls out.
11. Layer tomato onto every tart and set apart for a second.
12. Slice 1/2 medium onion thin, then caramelize the onion and 2 tsp. Minced garlic in 2 tbsp. Olive oil.
13. Add caramelized onions and garlic on top of the tomato.
14. Disintegrate goat cheese and sprinkle clean thyme over each tart, then bake for an additional 5 to 6 mins or until the cheese starts to soften.
15. Serve heat!

o   This makes a complete of 12 Goat Cheese Tomato cakes. each tart comes out to 162 cals, 15.6g fat, 2.1g carbs, and 2.8g protein.

24.   CAPRESE SALAD
SNACKS

INGREDIENTS:

- 1 CLEAN TOMATO
- 6 OZ. FRESH MOZZARELLA CHEESE
- 1/4 CUP CLEAN BASIL, CHOPPED
- 3 TBSP. OLIVE OIL
- SPARKLING CRACKED BLACK PEPPER
- KOSHER SALT

INSTRUCTIONS:

1. In a food processor, pulse chopped sparkling basil leaves with 2 tbsp. Olive Oil to make the Basil Paste.
2. Slice tomato into 1/four slices. You should be able to get at least 6 slices from the tomato.
3. cut Mozzarella into 1 ounces. Slices.
4. gather caprese salad by means of layering tomato, mozzarella, and basil paste.
5. Season with salt, pepper, and further olive oil. optionally available: reduce balsamic vinegar for balsamic reduction (be cautious of carb be counted).

o   This could make 2 servings total. Each serving has 405 cals, 36g fat, 4.5g carbs, and 15.5g protein.

25.   CHEESY BACONS
SNACKS

INGREDIENTS:

- EIGHT OZ.. MOZZARELLA CHEESE
- FOUR TBSP. ALMOND FLOUR
- FOUR TBSP. BUTTER, MELTED
- 3 TBSP. PSYLLIUM HUSK POW to DER
- 1 LARGE EGG
- 1/4 TSP. SALT
- 1/4 TSP. CLEAN GROUND BLACK PEPPER
- 1/8 TSP. GARLIC POWDER
- 1/8 TSP. ONION POWDER
- 10 SLICES SIR FRANCIS BACON
- 1 CUP OIL, LARD OR TALLOW
  (FOR FRYING)

INSTRUCTIONS:

1. Upload 4 ounces. (1/2) Mozzarella cheese to a bowl.
2. Microwave four tbsp. Butter for 15 to 20 seconds or till it's miles melted absolutely.
3. Microwave cheese for 45 to 60 seconds till melted and gooey (have to be a piece greater melted than shown in photograph).
4. Add 1 egg and butter to the mixture and mix well.
5. Upload four tbsp. Almond flour, three tbsp. Psyllium husk, and the relaxation of your spices to the mixture (1/4 tsp. Salt, 1/4 tsp. Clean floor Black pepper, 1/8 tsp. Garlic Powder, and 1/8 tsp. Onion Powder).
6. Blend everything together and sell off it out onto a silpat. Roll the dough out, or the use of your arms, shape dough right into a rectangle.
7. Spread the rest of the cheese over half of of the dough and fold the dough over lengthwise.

8. Fold the dough again vertically so that you form a rectangular shape.
9. Crimp the rims the usage of your arms and press the dough collectively right into a rectangle. You want the filling to be tight interior.
10. Using a knife, cut the dough into 20 squares.
11. Cut each slice of William Maxwell Aitken in half, then lay the rectangular on the stop of 1 piece of Sir Francis Bacon.
12. Roll the dough into the 1st baron beaverbrook tightly till the ends are overlapping. You could "stretch" your Baron Verulam in case you want to before rolling.
13. Use a toothpick to cozy the publisher 1st baron verulam after you roll it.
14. Do that for every piece of dough which you have. At the give up you may have 20 tacky William Maxwell Aitken bombs.
15. Warmness up oil, lard, or tallow to 350 to 375F and then fry the tacky 1st baron beaverbrook bombs three or four pieces at a time.
16. Take away to a paper towel to drain and cool as soon as finished.
17. Serve up!

o   This makes a complete of 20 tacky publisher 1st baron verulam Bombs. every comes out to be 89 cals, 7.2g fats, 0.6g carbs, and 5g protein.

26. CHIA SEED BLONDIES
SNACKS

INGREDIENTS:

2 1/4 CUPS PECANS, ROASTED
1/2 CUP CHIA SEEDS, GROUND
1/4 CUP BUTTER, MELTED
1/FOUR CUP ERYTHRITOL, POWDERED
3 TBSP. SF TORANI SALTED CARAMEL
10 DROPS LIQUID STEVIA
3 BIG EGGS
1 TSP. BAKING POWDER
3 TBSP. HEAVY CREAM
1 PINCH SALT

INSTRUCTIONS:

1. Preheat oven to 350f. Measure out 2 1/4 cup pecans (i order mine from amazon) and bake for about 10 mins. Once you can smell a nutty aroma, do away with nuts and set aside.
2. Grind half cup complete chia seeds in a spice grinder till a meal forms.
3. Get rid of chia meal and location in a bowl. Subsequent, grind 1/4 cup erythritol in a spice grinder till powdered. Set inside the identical bowl because the chia meal.
4. Location 2/three of roasted pecans in food processor.
5. Process nuts, scraping aspects down as wanted, until a clean nut butter is fashioned.
6. Upload three big eggs, 10 drops liquid stevia, 3 tbsp. Sf salted caramel torani syrup, and a pinch of salt to the chia combination. Blend this collectively properly.
7. Upload pecan butter to the batter and blend once more.
8. The use of a rolling pin, destroy the relaxation of the roasted pecans into chunks inside of a plastic bag.
9. Upload crushed pecans and 1/4 cup melted butter into the batter.

10. Blend batter properly, then add three tbsp. Heavy cream and 1 tsp. Baking powder. Blend the entirety collectively well.
11. Degree out the batter into a 9×9 tray and smooth out.
12. Bake for 20 minutes or until favored consistency.
13. Permit cool for about 10 mins. Slice off the rims of the brownie to create a uniform rectangular. That is what i call "the bakers deal with" – yep, you guessed it!
14. Snack on those terrible boys at the same time as you get them equipped to serve to anybody else. The so to known as "fine element" of the brownie are the rims, and that's why you should have it all.
15. Serve up and consume in your hearts (or as a substitute macros) content material!

o   This makes 16 overall Pecan Butter Chia Seed Blondies. each blondie comes out to 174 cals, 17.1g fats, 1.1g net carbs, and three.9g protein.

27.   AVOCADO LIME SORBET
SNACKS

INGREDIENTS:

- 2 MEDIUM HASS AVOCADOS
- 1/4 CUP NOW ERYTHRITOL, POWDERED
- 2 MEDIUM LIMES, JUICED & ZESTED
- 1 CUP COCONUT MILK (FROM CARTON)
- 1/4 TSP. LIQUID STEVIA
- 1/4 HALF CUP CILANTRO, CHOPPED

INSTRUCTIONS:

1. Slice avocados in half of. Use the butt of a knife and force it into the pits of the avocados. Slowly twist and pull knife until placed is removed.
2. Slice avocado half of vertically via the flesh, making approximately five slices in step with 1/2 of an avocado. Use a spoon to carefully

scoop out the pieces. Relaxation portions on foil and squeeze juice of half of lime over the tops.

3. Keep avocado in freezer for at least three hours. Simplest begin the subsequent step 2 half of hours once you positioned the avocado in the freezer.
4. The use of a spice grinder, powder 1/4 cup NOW Erythritol until a confectioner's sugar sort of consistency is performed.
5. In a pan, carry 1 cup Coconut Milk (from Carton) to a boil.
6. Zest the two limes you've got at the same time as coconut milk is heating up.
7. Once coconut milk is boiling, upload lime zest and continue to permit the milk reduce in volume.
8. When you see that the coconut milk is starting to thicken, put off and location into a box. It ought to have decreased through approximately 25%.
9. Keep the coconut milk combination in the freezer and allow it cool.
10. Chop 1/4 half cup cilantro, depending on how an awful lot cilantro taste you'd like.
11. Cast off avocados from freezer. They need to be absolutely frozen along with the lime juice. The lime juice need to have helped them no longer flip brown.
12. Upload avocado, cilantro, and juice from 1 half of lime into the meals processor. Pulse until a corpulent consistency is achieved.
13. Pour coconut milk aggregate over the avocados within the food processor. Upload 1/four tsp. Liquid Stevia to this.
14. Pulse mixture together till desired consistency is reached. This takes about 2 to 3 mins.
15. Go back to freezer to freeze, or serve right away!

○ This makes four overall servings of Cilantro Infused Avocado Lime Sorbet. Every serving comes out to 180 cals, 16g fats, 3.5g carbs, and 2g protein.

SNACKS

INGREDIENTS:

MAPLE BACON CAKE POPS

- 6 OZ..BURGERS' SMOKEHOUSE COUNTRY BACON
- 5 BIG EGGS, SEPERATED
- 1/4 CUP MAPLE SYRUP
- (RECIPE RIGHT HERE)
- HALF OF TSP. VANILLA EXTRACT
- 1/4 CUP NOW ERYTHRITOL
- 1/4 TSP. LIQUID STEVIA
- 1 CUP HONEYVILLE ALMOND FLOUR
- 2 TBSP. PSYLLIUM HUSK POWDER
- 1 TSP. BAKING POWDER
- 2 TBSP. BUTTER
- HALF TSP. CREAM OF TARTAR

SALTED CARAMEL GLAZE

- 5 TBSP. BUTTER
- 5 TBSP. HEAVY CREAM
- 2 HALF TBSP. TORANI SUGAR LOOSE SALTED CARAMEL

INSTRUCTIONS:

1. Slice 6 oz. Burgers' Smokehouse us of a Viscount St. Albans into small chew size chunks.
2. both freezing the publisher 1st baron verulam for 30 minutes prior, or using scissors usually helps with this process.
3. warmth a pan to medium high warmth and cook dinner the Bacon till crisp.

4. once crisp, put off the William Maxwell Aitken from the pan and permit to dry on paper towels. store excess Bacon grease to saute veggies or different meats in it.

5. Preheat oven to 325F. In 2 separate bowls, separate the egg yolks from the egg whites of 5 large eggs.

6. within the bowl with the egg yolks, add 1/four cup maple syrup (recipe right here), 1/four cup erythritol, 1/4 tsp. liquid stevia, and 1/2 tsp. vanilla extract.

7. the use of a hand mixer, mix this together for approximately 2 minutes. The egg yolks must turn out to be lighter in colour.

8. upload 1 cup Honeyville almond flour, 2 tbsp. psyllium husk powder, 2 tbsp. butter, and 1 tsp. baking powder.

9. mix this once more till a thick batter form.

10. Wash off the whisks of the hand mixer in the sink to ensure all traces of fats are washed off of the whisks.

11. upload half of tsp. cream of tartar to the egg whites.

12. Whisk the egg whites using a hand mixer until solid peaks form.

13. add 2/three crisped Francis Bacon into the cake pop batter.

14. upload about 1/3 of the egg whites into the batter and aggressively mix together.

15. The batter need to be a lot less dry now. upload the rest of the egg whites and lightly fold them in to the batter.

16. The end result ought to be a mild and airy batter.

17. Spoon mixture into a greased cake pop pan (i take advantage of this one from Nordic Ware), filling with a mound of batter that rises above the mildew. area the lid on top and bake for 20 to 25 minutes. you could both make 24 more cake pops, or make cupcakes with the remaining batter (identical cook time, yields about 7 cupcakes).

18. as soon as finished, take away the cake pops and permit cool.

19. as the cake pops are cooling, we want to make the sauce. you can either make this in 3 batches (as you will the cake pops) or you may make it into 1 large batch. I choose to do it three times. add butter to the pan over medium to low warmth and cook.

20. cook dinner the butter till it's browned and the effervescent stops.

21. upload heavy cream and sugar free torani salted caramel syrup to the pan.

22. The cream ought to bubble proper away.

23. blend everything collectively and keep to prepare dinner it whilst letting it reduce some. as soon as you may pull your spoon thru the mixture and it slowly comes lower back together, that's when it's geared up.

24. Poke lollipop sticks thru the cake pops and dip into caramel sauce.

25. enjoy your meal!

o Serving comes with 36 total caramel glazed pops with 80 cals, 7g fats, 0.6g carbs, 31g protein.

29. COCONUT CREAM YOGURT
SNACKS

INGREDIENTS:

- 1 CAN COMPLETE FATS COCONUT MILK
- 2 DRUGS NOW PROBIOTIC to 10
- HALF OF TSP. NOW XANTHAN GUM (1/4 TSP. SPLIT AMONG BOTH JARS)
- 2/3 CUP HEAVY WHIPPING CREAM
- TOPPINGS OF YOUR PREFERENCE

INSTRUCTIONS:

1. Open a can of coconut milk and stir it nicely. You need to make certain the cream and water in the can is very well mixed.
2. put the coconut milk into some thing box you'd like. I seperated mine into 2 200mL mason jars. Have your NOW Probiotic to 10 handy.
3. turn your oven mild on and location the jars in the oven. close the oven door, keeping the light on, and allow it take a seat for 12 to 24 hours overnight. The longer the bacteria can way of life, the thicker the combination gets, but it doesn't make too large of a difference.
4. Empty all of your yogurt into a blending bowl and sprinkle 1/2 tsp. Xanthan gum over it. using a hand mixer, mix this nicely.
5. In a separate bowl, whip up 2/three cup heavy cream till stiff peaks shape. You need this to be strong cream almost.
6. sell off the stable cream into the yogurt and mix on a low speed until the consistency you want is completed.
7. add toppings, flavorings, or fillings of your choice and enjoy!

o   ½ cup per serving with 315 cals, 31.3 g fats, 4.3g carbs, and 0g protein.

30.   PROSCIUTTO WRAPPED SHRIMP

SNACKS

INGREDIENTS:

- 10 OZ. PRE COOKED SHRIMP
- 11 SLICES PROSCIUTTO
- 1/THREE CUP BLACKBERRIES, FLOOR
- 1/THREE CUP CRIMSON WINE
- 2 TBSP. OLIVE OIL
- 1 TBSP. MINT LEAVES, CHOPPED
- 1 TO 2 TBSP. NOW ERYTHRITOL
- (TO TASTE)

INSTRUCTIONS:

1. Preheat your oven to 425F. Slice prosciutto in half of or in thirds, depending on what number of shrimp you have got and their length. Wrap shrimp in prosciutto, starting from the tail and working your manner up. Lay on a baking sheet, drizzle with 2 tbsp. olive oil, and prepare dinner for 15 minutes.
2. In a spice grinder, grind 1/three cup Blackberries.
3. In a pan, add the blackberry puree and mint leaves. add 1 to 2 tbsp. erythritol, to your tastes, then let cook for 2 to 3 mins.

4. upload 1/3 cup purple wine to the sauce and blend properly. Then let reduce beneath simmer. flavor when reduced and upload extra sweetener if wanted.
5. Serve with sauce on the aspect or drizzled over!

○ Comes with 4 servings each with 247 cals, 12.8g fats, 1g carbs, 13.8g protein.

31. DE CRÈME POTS
SNACKS

INGREDIENTS:

- 1 1/2 CUP HEAVY CREAM
- 1/4 CUP NOW ERYTHRITOL (POWDERED)
- 1/4 TSP. LIQUID STEVIA
- 1/4 TSP. SALT
- FOUR BIG EGG YOLKS
- 6 TBSP. WATER
- 1 TBSP. MAPLE SYRUP
- (SUB IN 1 TSP. MAPLE EXTRACT + 1/4 TSP. XANTHAN GUM IF YOU'D LIKE)
- 1/2 TSP. VANILLA EXTRACT
- 1 TSP. MAPLE EXTRACT

INSTRUCTIONS:

1. Preheat your oven to 300F. begin through separating the yolks of four eggs and setting them apart. you may keep the whites to feature to extraordinary cake recipes across the web site.
2. the use of a spice grinder (you could pick this one up reasonably to priced), powder 1/four cup NOW erythritol. Be careful when you take the lid off because powder will drift into the air.
3. blend the powdered erythritol with 6 tbsp. water in a small saucepan.
4. blend together 1 1/2 cups heavy cream, 1/4 tsp. liquid stevia, 1/4 tsp. salt, half tsp. vanilla extract, and 1 tsp. maple extract in a larger saucepan.
5. brilliant both of the mixtures to a rolling boil. as soon as the cream reaches a boil, stir vigorously and flip heat down to low. from time to time stir this as you figure with the other combination.

6. once the water and erythritol has been boiling for a minute, upload 1 tbsp. ma to ple syrup. in case you don't need to make the complete maple syrup recipe for 1 tbsp., you're welcome to sub in 1 tsp. Maple Extract + 1/4 tsp. Xanthan Gum in case you'd like.
7. Whisk egg yolks well with a whisk till lighter in coloration.
8. retain boiling the water and erythritol combination till it has reduced some and a watery syrup is formed.
9. Pour the water and erythritol combination into the heavy cream and stir to com to bine.
10. Slowly pour 1/four of the cream combination into the egg yolks at the same time as blending. You need to mood the egg yolks so make sure you add slowly and no longer too much right now.
11. degree out the combination between 4 or 6 ramekins relying on the scale of the ramekin.
12. Fill baking sheet 2/3 of the way with water. placed your ramekins in the water and bake at 300F for 40 minutes.
13. Take out of the oven and allow cool for 10 to 15 minutes. You cannot refrigerate them in case you'd like them to be greater of a mild custard or pudding texture. you may devour them warm for a velvety tender and easy texture.
14. who're we kidding? Serve them up!

- This made 4 servings, however you're welcome to divide them into smaller servings. each serving 359 cals, 34.9g fat, 3g carbs, and a pair of.8g Protein.

32.   BUTTER CHIA SQUARES

SNACKS

INGREDIENTS:

HALF OF CUP RAW ALMONDS
1 TBSP. + 1 TSP. COCONUT OIL
FOUR TBSP. NOW ERYTHRITOL
2 TBSP. BUTTER
1/FOUR CUP HEAVY CREAM
1/4 TSP. LIQUID STEVIA
1 HALF OF TSP. VANILLA EXTRACT
1/2 CUP UNSWEETENED SHREDDED COCONUT FLAKES
1/FOUR CUP CHIA SEEDS
1/2 CUP COCONUT CREAM
2 TBSP. COCONUT FLOUR

INSTRUCTIONS:

1. Add half cup uncooked Almonds to a pan and toast for approximately 7 minutes on medium low warmness. Just sufficient so you start to smell the nuttiness popping out.
2. Add the nuts to the food processor and grind them.
3. Once they attain a mealy consistency, upload 2 tbsp. NOW Erythritol and 1 tsp. Coconut Oil.
4. Keep grinding almonds until almond butter is fashioned.
5. In a pan, melt 2 tbsp. Butter on medium warmness whilst stirring. Do this until the butter is browned.
6. As soon as butter is browned, upload 1/4 cup Heavy Cream, 2 tbsp. NOW Erythritol, 1/4 tsp. Liquid Stevia, and 1 1/2 tsp. Vanilla Extract to the butter. Flip heat to low and stir nicely because the cream bubbles.
7. Grind 1/four Cup Chia Seeds in a spice grinder till a powder is formed.

8. Begin toasting chia seeds and 1/2 Cup Unsweetened Shredded Coconut Flakes in a pan on medium low. You need the coconut to just slightly brown.
9. Add almond butter to the butter and heavy cream combination and stir it in nicely. Let it prepare dinner down right into a paste.
10. In a square (or something size you need) baking dish, add the almond butter aggregate, toasted chia and coconut combination, and 1/2 Cup Coconut Cream. You could add the coconut cream to a pan to melt it slightly earlier than adding it.
11. Upload 1 tbsp. Coconut oil and a couple of tbsp. Coconut Flour and blend the whole thing to to gether properly.
12. The use of your arms, percent the combination into the baking dish properly.
13. Refrigerate combination for at least an hour and then take it out of the baking dish. It should keep shape now.
14. Chop the combination into squares or any shape you'd like and put again within the fridge for at least a few greater hours. You can use excess aggregate to shape greater squares, but I ate it as a substitute.
15. Take out and snack on it as you want!

- o This makes 14 total Almond Butter Chia Squares. per square, it's miles 120 carbs, 11.1g fats, 1.4g carbs, and 2.4g Protein. That's 83% fats, 5% carbs, and 8% protein.

33.   LIME CHEESECAKES
SNACKS

INGREDIENTS:

CHEESECAKE CRUST

- 1/2 CUP MACADAMIA NUTS
- HALF CUP HONEYVILLE ALMOND FLOUR
- 1/4 CUP BLOODLESS BUTTER
- 1/4 CUP NOW ERYTHRITOL
- 1 HUGE EGG YOLK

KEY LIME FILLING

- EIGHT OZ. CREAM CHEESE
- 1/4 CUP BUTTER
- 1/4 CUP NOW ERYTHRITOL
- 1/4 TSP. LIQUID STEVIA
- 1 TO 2 TBSP. KEY LIME JUICE (ABOUT 2 KEY LIMES FRESH IS EXCEPTIONAL)
- 2 HUGE EGGS
- ZEST OF TWO KEY LIMES

INSTRUCTIONS:

1. Preheat your oven to 350F. In a food processor, add the 1/2 cup of macadamia nuts.
2. Grind the nuts into a rough meal consistency, then add 1/four cup of NOW erythritol.
3. Pulse for some moments after which upload 1/2 Cup Honeyville almond flour. Pulse once more until all is mixed.
4. Dice 1/4 cup bloodless butter and upload that into the food processor. Pulse once more until the mixture begins to clump.
5. Upload 1 egg yolk and pulse again until all the dough clumps.
6. Eliminate the dough from the meals processor and knead together together with your hands.
7. Using some silicone cupcake molds (or just a ordinary greased cupcake tin), fill the wells approximately 1/8 to one/four of the way complete. This depends on how thick you want your crust. In case you make the crust skinny, you may be able to make extra cheesecake cupcakes.
8. Bake the crust for 5 to 7 mins at 350F. They shouldn't be browned while you are taking them out, they will look greasy and undercooked.
9. Even as the crust is cooking, beat collectively 1 block of cream cheese (eight ounces.) and 1/four cup butter.
10. As soon as the butter and cream cheese is mixed, upload the 2 eggs and blend again.
11. Upload 1/4 Cup NOW erythritol and 1/4 tsp. Liquid stevia then mix once more.
12. Ultimately, upload the zest of approximately 2 key limes and the juice from 2 (this is approximately 2 Tbsp. Of juice). Blend once more until absolutely mixed.
13. Once the crusts are out of the oven, let them cool for 3 to five minutes and then pour the aggregate into the molds. Fill them so they depart a few space on the top because they may upward push as they cook dinner and can spill over.
14. Bake the cheesecakes for 30 to 35 minutes at 350F.
15. Cool the cheesecakes for 20 to 30 minutes after which save within the fridge in a single day.
16. Add a few more key lime zest over the top and serve!

- This makes 12 total Key Lime Cheesecakes. Every cheesecake has 226 cals, 20.8g fat, 2.2g carbs, and 4.2g Protein

34.   BUCKEYE COOKIES

SNACKS

INGREDIENTS:

- 2 HALF CUPS HONEYVILLE ALMOND FLOUR
- HALF CUP PEANUT BUTTER
- 1/4 CUP COCONUT OIL
- 1/4 CUP NOW ERYTHRITOL
- 3 TBSP. MAPLE SYRUP (RECIPE RIGHT HERE)
- 1 TBSP. VANILLA EXTRACT
- 1 HALF TSP. BAKING POWDER
- HALF OF TSP. SALT
- 2 TO 3 CHOCOPERFECTION BARS (OR 3 TO 4 SQUARES 90%+ DARK CHOCOLATE)

INSTRUCTIONS:

1. In a large blending bowl, upload half of Cup Peanut Butter, 1/four Cup Coconut Oil, three Tbsp. Maple Syrup (recipe right here), and 1 Tbsp. Vanilla Extract.
2. In a seperate bowl, upload 2 half Cups Honeyville Almond Flour, 1/4 Cup NOW Erythritol, 1 1/2 tsp. Baking Powder, and half tsp. Salt.
3. The use of a hand mixer, mix together the wet elements.
4. Sift the dry components into the wet substances the use of a colander or sifter.
5. Mix everything together until it paperwork a crumbled dough.
6. The usage of your palms, blend together all the dough into a ball. Wrap in plastic wrap and refrigerate for half to hour.

7. Earlier than getting your dough out, split 2 Chocoperfection (or 90%+ dark Chocolate) bars into small chunks. You want to in shape 1 to 2 portions into each cookie.
8. Preheat your oven to 350F. Then, rip off small chunks of dough at a time.
9. Press the chocolate into the dough.
10. Seal the dough together with your palms till the chocolate can't be visible.
11. Press the dough into a rounded tablespoon for constant cookies.
12. Lay all cookies down on a silpat approximately 1 inch faraway from every different. You need to get 20 cookies.
13. Bake cookies for 15 to 18 minutes. Optional: Broil cookies for added 2 to 3 minutes to brown the tops.
14. Let cool and serve!

- This makes 20 total cookies. Each cookie is 148 cals, 13.6g fats, 2.5g net carbs, and four.4g protein. A great keto snack!

35.   SESAME LEMON CAKE

SNACKS

INGREDIENTS:

BASE

- 1 BIG EGG
- 2 TBSP. BUTTER
- 2 TBSP. HONEYVILLE ALMOND FLOUR
- HALF TSP. BAKING POWDER

FLAVOR

- 1 TBSP. SESAME SEED • 1 TSP. LEMON JUICE
- 1/FOUR TSP. CUMIN
- 1/FOUR TSP. PEPPER
- PINCH SALT

INSTRUCTIONS:

1. Get your mug ready! Very well, I'm the use of a cup for this one. Upload 1 huge Egg, 2 Tbsp. Honeyville Almond Flour, 2 Tbsp. Of Room Temperature Butter, 1 Tbsp.
2. Sesame Seed, 1 tsp. Lemon Juice, 1/2 tsp. Baking Powder, 1/4 tsp. Cumin, 1/four tsp. Black Pepper, and a pinch of salt.
3. Microwave this for 75 seconds on excessive (strength level 10). Then, gently slam your cup in opposition to a plate so that it comes out of the mug (or cup in this example).
4. Pinnacle with extra sesame seeds and lemon .

o Per serving this is 412 energy, 37g fats, 3g net Carbs, and 11g Protein.Of path, you could usually cut up that in half of if you could't come up with the money for that many energies! Or, you could update an entire meal with this. Whats up new meal!

36. COUNTRY GRAVY
SIDES

INGREDIENTS:

- FOUR OZ.. BREAKFAST SAUSAGE
- 2 TBSP. BUTTER
- 1 CUP HEAVY CREAM
- 1/2 TSP. GUAR GUM
- SALT AND PEPPER TO TASTE

INSTRUCTIONS:

1. Add sausage to the pan and permit brown on all sides.
2. Put off sausage from the pan, but hold as much fat in there as viable.
3. Add 2 tbsp. Butter to the pan and let it soften.
4. As soon as butter is absolutely melted, add heavy cream to the pan. Stir it because it bubbles.
5. Upload the guar gum to the pan and stir vigorously whilst the cream is bub to bling. Permit the combination thicken to the factor in which you could run your spatula thru it and it's going to take a moment to shut the gap.
6. Add sausage back into the pan and stir collectively. Serve and experience! Oh, and don't forget to test out keto delivered if you need keto candies on your doorstep every month!

- o This makes a complete of four servings of 10 Minute Keto united states Gravy. each serving comes out to be 346 cals, 38g fat, 1.5g carbs, and 4g protein.

37.   MUSHROOM RICE PILAF

SIDES

INGREDIENTS:

- 1 CUP HEMP SEEDS
- 2 TBSP. BUTTER
- THREE MEDIUM MUSHROOMS
- 1/4 CUP SLICED ALMONDS
- 1/2 CUP CHOOK BROTH
- 1/2 TSP. GARLIC POWDER
- 1/4 TSP. DRIED PARSLEY
- SALT AND PEPPER TO FLAVOR

INSTRUCTIONS:

1. Wash and slice mushrooms into small chunks.
2. Upload butter to a pan over medium heat and permit melt and bubble. Once bub to bling, add sliced almonds and mushrooms to the pan.
3. As soon as mushrooms are smooth, add hemp seeds to the pan. Blend together properly.
4. Add chook broth and seasoning to the pan and stir collectively nicely. Flip down the warmth to medium low and allow the chook broth simmer and be absorbed.
5. When you're satisfied with the consistency, turn the pan off and dish out!
6. This goes tremendous with fowl dishes, but may be used with almost some thing.

- o This makes a complete of four servings of Keto Mushroom Wild Rice Pilaf. Each serving comes out to be 325 cals, 26.3g fat, 1.3g carbs, and 14.8g protein.

38. CREAMED SPINACH
SIDES

INGREDIENTS:

- 10 OZ.. FROZEN SPINACH
- THREE TBSP. PARMESAN CHEESE
- 3 TBSP. CREAM CHEESE
- 2 TBSP. BITTER CREAM
- 1/4 TSP. GARLIC POWDER
- 1/4 TSP. ONION POWDER
- SALT AND PEPPER TO FLAVOR

INSTRUCTIONS:

1. Defrost frozen spinach in the microwave until warmed thru, normally about 6 to 7 minutes.
2. Heat a pan on the range to medium to excessive warmness. As soon as the pan is warm, add the spinach and permit some of the water boil off. Season the spinach right here and blend together.
3. Add cream cheese and stir together till cream cheese is melted.
4. Upload bitter cream and mix together. Flip the pan down to low heat at this point.
5. Eventually, add parmesan cheese and stir until the creamed spinach thickens.
6. Serve up! It is going top notch with just about something!

- This makes a total of 3 servings of easy Keto Creamed Spinach.every serving comes out to be 157 cals, 13.3g fat, 2g net carbs, and 5.7g protein.

- This makes 2 general servings of Fried Kale Sprouts. every serving comes out to be 109 cals, 8.5g fat, 1.5g carbs, and 4g protein.

Lightning Source UK Ltd.
Milton Keynes UK
UKHW020637080721
386832UK00012B/1186